Hypertension

The Ultimate Information Guide for Hypertension

Hypertension Facts, Diagnosis, Symptoms, Treatment, Causes, Effects, Unconventional Treatments, and More!

By Frederick Earlstein

Foreword

The medical term itself seems innocuous enough, but hypertension is one the deadliest, silent serial killer diseases which has consistently taken lives. We see recently that more and more casualties have fallen victim to this silent malady which has plagued seemingly "healthy" people, young and old.

Hypertension does not choose its victims. The "victims" of this dreaded disease are either susceptible to the diseases either by the lifestyle they lead or because of other diseases which may bring about this deadly killer of many. This book aims to enlighten the reader of the effects and pitfalls of hypertension and help lower the number of incidences victims who die because of increased high blood pressure.

Table of Contents

Introduction

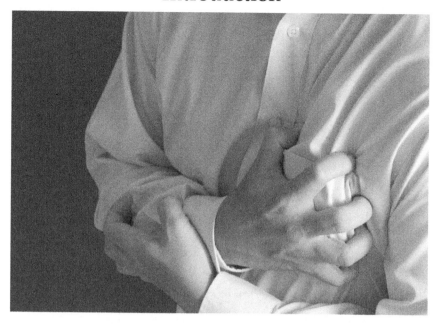

The World Health Organization, or WHO, has suggested that the prevalence of processed foods, with its high amounts of salt, as the culprit in the increase of incidences of hypertension in humans all over the globe. In the United States alone the number of people with hypertension is around 85 million and rising.

Factors such as stress can cause and induce elevated levels of blood pressure. However, hypertension can also result from other conditions such as kidney disease. When undetected, untreated and unmanaged, hypertension can lead to a stroke, heart attack and other medical conditions.

But let's not get ahead of ourselves and allow us to delve in deeper into and identify causes of this long term medical condition to know what we can do to avoid it, maintain it and treatments available.

What is Hypertension?

Hypertension, or its abbreviation HTN or HT, is also widely known in layman's terms as high blood pressure (HBP). Hypertension is a silent yet for the most part a dangerous medical condition wherein a person's blood pressure in their arteries is constantly increased or elevated. High blood pressure typically does not display symptoms until it is bothersome for the individual most especially for those whose lifestyles make themselves prone to the disease. Other times, genetics play a big role in the incidence of hypertension in a person. Long term high blood pressure (HBP) is a critical and major risk indication of brain damage that can lead to stroke or other neurological illnesses, cardiovascular diseases like a coronary artery, loss of vision, peripheral vascular disease, and renal diseases.

There are two classifications of high blood pressure which claim lives every year. The first sort of HBT is what medical experts call primary, or essential, high blood pressure. Genetic and lifestyle factors make up 90-95% of the total number of people with this condition increasing the risk of HBT for people with poor lifestyle choices.

Maintaining a lifestyle of excessive drinking, smoking, too much salt intake and poor dietary practices, factoring in environmental stressors as well are some of the major causes of HBT which leads to hypertension.

Secondary high blood pressure make up for the remaining 5-10% of the population of people with hypertension. Secondary high blood pressure is due to other factor identifiable like an endocrine disorder, the use of birth control pills, chronic kidney disease and the narrowing of kidney arteries.

Medications and lifestyle changes make a big impact on the lowering of blood pressure and assist greatly in decreasing the dangers of health complications due to hypertension. Changing one's lifestyle includes losing weight, dramatically lessening the intake of salt, maintaining a regular exercise regimen and thoughtfully and truthfully looking at one's dietary choices and making drastic changes to eat healthier. In fact, 90% of people with hypertension are able to control the condition using any of the three available medications in the market presently. Moderately high arterial blood pressure, which is defined as >160/100 mmHg is treated and has been successfully responsible for improved life expectancy in many patients as well. However, the efficiency of treatment of blood pressure between 140/90 mmHg and 160/100 mmHg is still unclear. There has been a contradiction in the benefits of treatment with some reporting of positive results and benefits whilst others see little to no positive, beneficial evidence.

The global number of individuals affected by high blood pressure is at a staggering range between 16 and 37%. Hypertension was said to have been the culprit of deaths around the world in 2010, making up 18% of fatalities due and related to hypertension.

High Blood vs. Low Blood

Let's discuss the key difference between both high and low pressures. High Blood Pressure (HBT) and Low Blood Pressure (LBT) are two varied conditions which happen when blood pressure levels are not at normal acceptable ranges.

Both medical names are suggestive conditions of the health situation of the patient. High blood pressure is what we call it when a person's blood pressure reading is usually and consistently too high. Alternatively, low blood pressure suggests of blood pressure readings which are usually too low. Both these conditions entail each their own symptoms, dangers and medication and/or treatments.

BP, or blood pressure, refers basically to the blood pressure in the bloodstream. It basically defines that the pressure which the blood exerts against the walls of the vein or artery. There is a twofold measurement of the blood which is the systolic pressure and the diastolic pressure.

The pressure in the veins or arteries when the heart beats and fills them with blood is systolic pressure. The pressure in the veins when the heart is at rest between beats is what is called the diastolic pressure. Both these pressures are measured with an instrument bearing a blood pressure cuff and are called a sphygmomanometer. Both high blood and low blood pressures (HBP and LBP) are two different types of conditions which happen when the blood pressure of a patient or individual is not at proper and health-acceptable situations.

Hypertension by the Numbers

In the United States alone, the number of physician visits related to high blood pressure and hypertension is at an extreme high with 39.9 billion people having been diagnosed with essential hypertension. This accounts for the number of people who need to make wiser choices in their diet, and lifestyles. On the other hand, there are at least 3.7 million people who have visited hospitals as outpatients and have been diagnosed with essential hypertension, bringing up the risk to many more. The mortality rate of essential hypertension and hypertensive renal disease comes to 30, 221. 9 out of 100,000 of the population die of essential hypertension as well as hypertensive renal disease.

Looking outside of the United States borders, it has been determined that 7.5 million deaths are due to raised blood pressure and makes up for about 12.8% of the total sum of mortalities due to essential hypertension. This gives us a clear picture of disability adjusted life years or DALY and which accounts for 57 million individuals, about 3.7% of disability adjusted life years in all. Increased blood pressure puts an individual at a greater risk to have an ischemic or hemorrhagic stroke as well as coronary heart disease.

Upon investigation and years of medical observation and studies, it is the pressure levels of the blood which has historically and continuously been related to exposure and susceptibility of an individual to coronary heart disease and stroke. The dangers of cardiovascular disease in particular age groups doubles with each increment 20/10 mmHg of blood pressure, beginning at a low of 115/75 mmHg. Adding to stroke and coronary heart disease, raised blood pressure complications are also responsible for heart failure, renal impairment, peripheral vascular disease, visual impairment and retinal hemorrhage. A reduction in cardiovascular complications has been associated with treating systolic blood pressure and diastolic blood pressure until both come to less than 140/90 mmHg.

In 2008, the overall global occurrence of raised blood pressure in adults aged 25 years and above was noted to be a staggering 40%. It is to be said that between 1980 to 2008, the proportion of the global populace with uncontrolled hypertension and high blood pressure modestly during that period. But because of ageing and population growth a spike in the number of individuals was noted. From 600 million people in 1980 to 1 billion people in 2008, shows how much hypertension and its effects affect the global population.

Amongst regions where the World Health Organization if present, the occurrence and persistence of incidences of people with high blood pressure were highest in Africa accounting for 46% for males and females combined. Raised blood pressure also account for both men and women, with prevalence rates that are over 40%.

In the World Health Organizations areas of the Americas, it was noted that the lowest prevalence was recorded at 35% for both males and females. The males in this area were likelier to have higher prevalence than women with numbers showing 39% of hypertensive men and 32% for women.

Collectively, in all World Health Organization areas, it has been determined that women have a lower prevalence than men to have increased blood pressure, and this data was only significant statistically in Europe and the Americas.

Blood Pressure Mechanics

Now that we have taken a look into the numbers and found out how much of a menace this silent killer is in the US and around the world, let's look at a handy table which gives us an idea of blood pressure readings and what they mean. This is a table of the blood pressure ranges as defined by the American Heart Association.

Systolic Diastolic

Normal BP	120	80
Prehypertension	ranges between 120 - 139	ranges between 80 - 89
Hypertension *stage 1	ranges between 140 - 159	ranges between 90 - 99
Hypertension *stage 2	160	100

Hypertensive Crisis	180	110

The human body is a marvelous machine with intricate workings that serve us well if we are mindful about avoiding what can be destructive to it, most times. We are given a certain extent of control over it that thoughtful care allows us to avoid some diseases and medical conditions to occur within it.

Primary hypertension is one such condition. Our veins require a certain amount of blood pressure of around 80 mmHg when at rest so that oxygen and important nutrients are able to reach where they need to be and this is the diastolic pressure which is the lower value. Not being able to allow oxygen and nutrients to travel where they must our arteries becomes as useless as used straws. Our arteries work much like a water hose needing some sort of constant pressure to make liquid within traverse.

Our heart, save for our brain is one amazing machine in its own making sure that the proper amounts of oxygen and nutrients are dispersed accordingly throughout our body even going against the force of gravity. You may recall that science classes in school liken our hearts to a pump which collects only the most essential blood amounts and pushing it out into the system of pipes by way of contracting its muscles and squeezing out the blood. This point of contraction exerted by the heart muscles is the higher value of the blood pressure reading and what is called the systolic pressure. The statistic benchmark for systolic pressure is at 120 mmHg.

A person's blood pressure gives a different reading throughout the day. BP reading is reading when a person is asleep and spikes when awake. There are situations which can affect our BP and may show a temporary rise when under stressful situations even in a healthy individual. This is why it is recommended to take a few readings in a span of a few minutes apart.

When taking your own blood pressure readings be sure to do it after you have rested. Avoid taking your BP after any strenuous activity - even waling up a flight of stairs can radically give you false reading. Should your reading be on the high side and display a reading of hypertensive crisis, take two to three minutes to rest and repeat the procedure. However, if a high reading of 180 over 110 persists even after rest is an indication of a risk of hypertension and will require medical attention immediately.

Chapter One: Hypertension and You

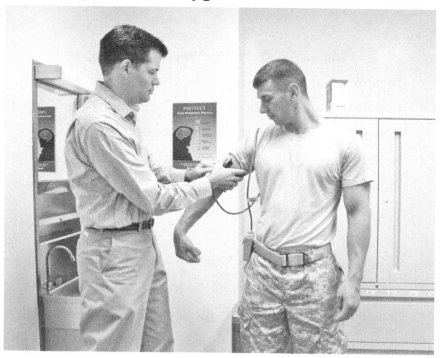

How can we tell if we are susceptible to hypertension or, worse, already suffer from it? With so much uncertainty around us, it should help to know that there are some things over which we have some control. Yes, it's true that is not always something consistently present in our lives, but there are some areas where we can work on to be able to live better, healthier lives. There are a number of factors which put individuals at risk for developing hypertension. Aside from leading an unhealthy lifestyle, age comes into factor for tendency of developing primary or essential hypertension for people over 60 years old. Blood pressure can increase incrementally because of the arteries stiffening up and narrowing down due to the buildup of plaque.

Ethnicity also comes into play with regard to hypertension development. The risk of developing hypertension is equally the same for both male and females; however men have notably been more prone to hypertension even at a young age. On the other hand increase in susceptibility for women increase as a female matures.

Let's delve in a little more to discover and identify factors that make people prone to hypertension. We want to reveal how to detect if this mute killer with little indication can in fact be detected or if there are signs that would give rise to concern about having the condition.

When do I have Hypertension?

Hypertension is not always apparent nor is it usually accompanied by visible symptoms, and is typically identified through screening. Most people with the condition are made aware of having the condition or when they seek healthcare for a physical issue unrelated to hypertension. There are a few individuals with high blood pressure that report headaches particularly describing the location of the pain at the back of the head and during the morning.

Vertigo, lightheadedness, a buzzing or ringing in the ears - called tinnitus is also reported by other individual as well as a change in vision or episodes of fainting. However, these symptoms may also be associated with some sort of anxiety or a situation of duress rather than with high blood pressure itself.

What are the causes high blood pressures? Knowing the causes can make quite the difference to anyone who may suspect they could be prone to the condition. Hypertension comes in two sorts and each type is caused by different things.

Let's discuss Primary hypertension which is the most typical sort found in most individuals. Primary hypertension is also known as essential hypertension. This sort of hypertension is developed over a period of time giving hardly any signs of identifiable cause. Researchers are admittedly still quite unclear of what mechanisms cause blood pressure to slowly increase however; it is suspected that a combination of factors could play a role.

Amongst these factors include a person's genes. There are some individuals who are predisposed genetically to hypertension. This could happen because of genetic abnormalities or gene mutations which were passed down from parents to child.

Another factor is physical changes in your body. If a part of your body does not function properly or accurately as it should, you may start to experience challenges in and throughout your body which was normally not felt. One of those issues could be high blood pressure.

An example we can cite is transformation in kidney functions. It is surmised that transformations in kidney function can upset a person's natural balance of salts and fluid. The change in functionality may cause your body's blood pressure to increase. Other existing health conditions such as cardiovascular disease are also indicators and predictors of hypertension.

The choices we make on our daily lives play a big part in our overall wellness. As time passes, unhealthy lifestyle choices we make like lack or complete absence of physical activity and poor dietary choices can truly take a bad toll on an individual's body. Our lifestyle and the choices we make, like smoking, excessive drinking and constantly being in stressful situations can and may lead to weight issues. When a person is overweight or obese it increases a person's risk for hypertension.

Time to look at the other sort of hypertension called Secondary hypertension. Secondary hypertension frequently happens fast and can be a lot more serious than that of primary hypertension. There are several conditions which may cause secondary hypertension and these include obstructive sleep apnea, kidney disease, problems with an individual's thyroid, side effects of medications, congenital heart defects, alcohol abuse or chronic use, use of illegal drugs, adrenal gland problems, as well as certain endocrine tumor.

In a nutshell, high blood pressure which isn't caused by other conditions or diseases is called primary, or essential, hypertension. If it develops as a result of another medical condition, this is what is called secondary hypertension.

How do I Measure my Blood Pressure?

There are a few steps which are simple enough to do by yourself to help get an accurate blood pressure reading. The first thing you want to do is find a quiet place before taking your blood pressure.

- You also need to make certain that the sphygmomanometer you have has the proper size cuff. If you are not sure or if you find yourself stumped with a plethora of questions you want to talk to your healthcare provider before making a purchase. Your physician or a registered nurse can give you recommendations. You want to avoid finger and/or wrist monitors as these do not ensure an accurate blood pressure reading as well as a proper sphygmomanometer does.

- You want to roll up the sleeve on your left arm and take off clothing which has tight sleeves, if required. if you are right-handed it would be better to take your blood pressure from your left arm.

- You need to take a load off and rest by sitting on a chair beside a table for at least 5 to 10 minutes with your left arm comfortably resting at a level with your heart. Remember how your mother or teacher barked at you to sit up straight? That is what you want to do with your back against the chair, with your legs uncrossed and feet squarely on the floor.

- You need to rest your forearm on the table positioning your arm so that you have the palm of your hand facing up. You must not talk, do anything else like read a newspaper, play video games or watch television during the process of taking your BP reading if you want an accurate one.

Let's now focus on taking your blood pressure accurately. When you purchase a sphygmomanometer, whether it is a manual or digital blood pressure monitor, first read then follow the instructions in the booklet mindfully.

The following steps provide an overview on how to take your blood pressure whether using either a manual or digital blood pressure monitor.

On a manual monitor:

- Find your pulse. Do this by lightly applying pressure to the crook of your arm - that is the inside bend of your elbow where the brachial artery is located. if you can't find your pulse then you may want to use a stethoscope, if you are using a manual monitor. If you are using a digital monitor then you may use the arm cuff in the area of your arm mentioned.

- Slip on the cuff onto your arm and make certain that the head of the stethoscope is resting over the brachial artery. The bottom part of the cuff should be about an inch over the crook of your elbow. Make sure that the fabric of the cuff if fastened securely on your arm but not too tightly.

- Place the earpieces of the stethoscope in your ears tilting the ear pieces ever so slightly forward to get the best sound results.

- When using a manual blood pressure device, you want to grip the pressure gauge in your left hand and the bulb on the other.

- Shut the airflow valve on the bulb of the device by turning the crew of the bulb clockwise.

- Proceed to inflate the cuff by squeezing the bulb. You will hear the sound of your pulse with the stethoscope.

- Mind the gauge of the monitor. Continue to inflate the cuff until you see the gauge read about 30 mmHg above the systolic pressure. You will not be able to hear your pulse at this point.

- Keep your eyes on the monitor gauge. Slowly let out the pressure in the cuff. Do this by turning the airflow valve counterclockwise.

- Still keeping your eyes on the gauge, the gauge should drop about 2 to 3 point with each heartbeat. You may have to practice doing this by turning the valve slowly. (Be patient. And if you feel insecure about making accurate readings, ask your practitioner if you are doing the procedure correctly).

- You want to listen carefully for the first beat. Once you hear it, take note of the number reading on the monitor - this is your systolic pressure; that is the exertion of the blood against the walls of your artery as your heart beats.

- Continue to deflate the cuff little by little.

- You want to listen until you do not hear the sound of your pulse. When you can no longer detect the sound of your pulse, take note of the reading on the gauge - this is your diastolic pressure or the pressure of your blood between heartbeats.

- You may proceed to deflate the cuff completely.

Things to take note of:

- Keep your arm held straight for the most accurate reading.

- Should you make a mistake and release pressure out too fast or perhaps was not able to locate of hear your pulse, remove the cuff, wait one minute, put it on again, and repeat the steps above.

On a digital monitor:

- Using your right hand, hold the bulb.

- Switch on the power button and all display symbols should briefly light up followed by a zero. This is an indication that the monitor is ready to use.

- Keep your eyes on the gauge. Inflate the cuff and continue doing so until you see the gauge read about 30 mmHg above your expected systolic pressure.

- Sit still and keep your eyes on the monitor. You should see the pressure reading show up on the screen. Values will appear on the screen.

- Wait for the long beep sound which signals the measurement is finished.

- Take note of the numbers on the screen. Systolic readings should appear on the left side of the screen and the diastolic pressure reading is on the right.

- Deflate the cuff.

Keep a record of your blood pressure readings. Keeping tabs on your blood pressure helps you monitor how your blood pressure fluctuates and differs from the time of the day. You want to take note of the date you took your blood pressure, the time of day when you did, the numbers of the systolic and diastolic readings, your heart rate as well as the arm which you used to take it. It would also be useful to jot down any events or situations which you may find useful for future reference. Taking down notes make it easier for you to relay information to your health care provider. It is also important specially if you are asked to take your blood pressure on a regular basis.

You should check the accuracy of the monitor you purchase at least once a year and bring it in with you to your doctor's office to make sure that it is giving you accurate results. This is carried out by making comparisons of your reading using your doctor's blood pressure monitor device and your machine.

Factors that Influences Blood Pressure Reading

Keep in mind that there are factors which influence your blood pressure to spike temporarily and should avoid to get proper and accurate reading. Some of these are cold temperatures, exercise, stress, smoking, caffeine and even some medicines. Try as best you can to avoid these before taking your blood pressure. You will also want to schedule specific times each day to take your blood pressure. Your medical practitioner may also request that you take your blood pressure readings a few times a day to help identify if it fluctuates.

Benefits of Home Blood Pressure Monitoring

Most doctors, if not all, make it a point to get a reading of your blood pressure with each visit. Diagnosing hypertension doesn't have to be complicated and is in fact as simple as taking your blood pressure reading routinely.

Should you have a high blood pressure reading, your physician may ask you to get more frequent readings over a period of a few days. Make sure to keep a tab on your readings by jotting them down on your little BP journal. Your doctor will need evidence which shows a sustained elevated reading before their patient is given a diagnosis of being hypertensive. Rarely is a hypertension diagnosis given after one reading.

Keep in mind that environmental factors could be affecting your blood pressure thereby giving varied results each time. You also need to remember that the levels of your blood pressure changes as the day wears on and you will need to be mindful about keeping a religious schedule. Set an alarm for each time of the day you have to monitor your blood pressure and veer not from those times each day.

Should your blood pressure consistently show a high reading, your physician will most likely request to have more tests carried out to rule out any other underlying conditions which may attribute to the high numbers of your blood pressure. These laboratory tests would likely include a cholesterol screening, a test of your heart's electrical activity and urine test. These tests are to help your physician any secondary underlying conditions which may be contributing to the elevation of your blood pressure.

Your doctor may likely to start treatment of your hypertension at this time. Your physician will want to give early treatment to reduce the likelihood of any further or lasting damage.

What is White Coat Hypertension?

Notice how your heart starts pounding at the thought of a looming visit to your dentist? This is also true for some individuals who are due for a physician visit. A visit to the doctor, for some is an experience ridden by inherent anxiety.

So there will be times when you get a high reading when your doctor does this simple procedure.

This is mostly all in the mind and the phenomenon is quite a real one for many, hence the term White Coat Hypertension. It is identified by high readings of your doctor but a relatively lower one when done in the comfort of your own home.

What is Labile Hypertension?

Labile hypertension is not to be mistaken for borderline hypertension. Labile hypertension is in fact what doctors call the condition of individuals who have frequent high or low blood pressure level changes. The condition is defined by a sudden onset and continuing fluctuation in an individual's blood pressure, which typically heighten from a normal, healthy blood pressure reading to a high blood pressure reading during varied times throughout the day.

There is a divide in the medical community about labile hypertension. Some see it as a faulty concept and, hence a faulty diagnosis whilst other see it as a condition which is treatable. Either way, labile hypertension is believed generally to have less clinical impact and significance on a patient as compared to the better understood condition called "fixed" hypertension.

Fixed hypertension is also a more dangerous condition. Guidelines for treatment of labile hypertension are vague and there are no accepted quantitative criteria to identify or understand the condition even though most physicians and health care providers are aware and know of the term. Nor are there guidelines for criteria of giving it as diagnosis.

What is Masked Hypertension?

Masked hypertension may happen to as much as 10% of the general population, and is crucial since masked hypertension is not diagnosed by regular medical exams, but it sums up to an adverse prognosis, either in terms of heightened target organ damage and cardiovascular episodes. It is identified as a normal blood pressure reading in the clinic or doctor's office of <140/90 mmHg, but a high blood pressure out of the clinic i.e. ambulatory daytime or home blood pressure >135/85 mmHg.

Some probable characteristics of patients who have masked hypertension are the following;

- male populace
- relatively young patient
- increased physical activities during daytime
- smoking habit

- drinking habit
- stress

Masked hypertension has also been identified in individuals and patients treated for hypertension. It was also described to have a worse prognosis than given from the clinic pressure in children in whom which masked hypertension could be the beginning of sustained hypertension.

Masked hypertension could be suspected in patients who have historically shown high blood pressure readings from time to time but who are normotensive when given a blood pressure reading in the clinic. This is why it is practical to keep a journal of your blood pressure readings, whether at your physician's clinic or at home.

Patients and individuals who display this should be monitored in and out of clinic. And this is when knowing how to take your own blood pressure reading accurately comes into play. Rather than dismissing these erratic readings, individuals of this sort should be encouraged to be more mindful about being vigilant of their blood pressure highs and lows. This goes for smokers and patients whose blood pressure is in the red or the pre-hypertensive range. The probable dangers of masked hypertension are extreme. However, the optimum strategy to detect this condition in the general population is yet to have better clarity.

Chapter Two: Effects, Causes, Signs and Symptoms

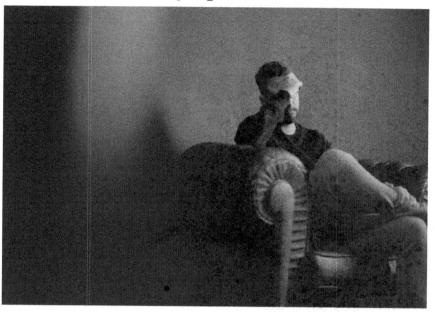

The sad truth is, many people suffer from the varied levels of hypertension and don't even know it. Many people succumb to this condition as they are not aware of the implications of either a pre-existing disease they may have such as thyroid problems, cardiovascular as well as kidney diseases or individuals leading unhealthy lifestyles who are not aware of the damage their habits and vices does on their physical well - being and health.

The effects of hypertension may be subtle, mimic other less alarming conditions and may be ignored. In fact, many have and the outcome of their fate depended on how soon this silent killer was detected. Sometimes, curbing this deadly condition is as simple as switching up one's lifestyle to one more conducive to health. Other times, medication is needed therefore a visit to the physician is imperative for those with pre-existing illnesses. Most of the time, patients who develop hypertension due to another disease has the advantage of being under a physician's care.

The moniker for hypertension, the "silent killer", is an apt one indeed since many patients with this condition are often oblivious to the symptoms they may display. As these exhibited signs are ignored, damage is caused to the internal organs like the kidneys. It also causes silent destruction to the cardiovascular system of the person.

The symptoms and signs of hypertension at any level can be elusively deceptive. Not only is your research now an important part of you getting back on the road to better health and improved wellness, this also allows you to become a proactive individual bent on living a better quality of life. In this chapter, we'll check out the effects of high blood pressure and what it does to an individual's body.

Effects of High Blood Pressure

As mentioned earlier, hypertension, or high blood pressure, can silently wreak havoc on your body for years before symptoms start manifesting. If left uncontrolled and unmaintained with physician care, medication or an altering of lifestyle, a person may end up with a disability, a very poor quality of life or worse, a killer heart attack. About half the populations of patients with undetected and untreated high blood pressure succumb to heart disease because of poor blood flow, also known as ischemic heart disease. Another third of these untreated patients are victims of sudden stroke.

The upside to this is that lifestyle changes coupled with treatment can control hypertension and lesson a person's risk of complications which are life threatening. Let's take a look at the complications high blood pressure brings about if not maintained and controlled.

Damage to a Person's Arteries

When arteries are in tip-top condition and healthy that means they are strong and elastic. The inner lining of the arteries are seamlessly smooth allowing blood to flow freely as it should. Healthy arteries are able to supply the proper amount of blood to important organs and tissues in our bodies with oxygen and nutrients.

Hypertension slowly increases the pressure of the blood which flows through one's arteries and as a result a person may develop narrowed and damaged arteries. Having high blood pressure may most likely slowly destroy the cells of your arteries inner lining. The fats in your diet, once it enters your bloodstream, can gather in the damaged artery walls and cause plaque buildup which in turn causes the arteries to become less and less flexible and elastic. When this occurs the blood flow through a person's body is limited.

Another frequent taker of lives is an aneurysm. As time passes and hypertension is not managed or detected in a patient, the constant and continuous pressure of blood coursing through a damaged and weakened artery can be cause for a section of the artery wall to become enlarged and form a bulge - this is an aneurysm. Aneurysms are able to form throughout a person's body, and within any artery, however, they are most commonly formed in the aorta, which is your body's biggest artery.

Damage to the Heart

Our heart is an amazing piece of organ responsible for pumping and supplying blood throughout your entire body. When high blood pressure remains uncontrolled it is cause for damage to a person's heart in a number of ways.

A coronary artery disease is a common damage to a person's heart with hypertension. It affects the arteries which are responsible for supplying blood to the muscles of the heart. When arteries are narrowed out by coronary artery disease this prevents the blood flow to freely course through a person's arteries. Needless to say, when blood supply cannot freely flow to the heart, an individual can feel chest pain, irregular heartbeats, called arrhythmias, or a heart attack.

Hypertension can cause an enlarged left heart. When high blood pressure forces an individual's heart to work harder than it needs to in order to supply and pump blood to the rest of the body this event makes the left ventricle of the individual's heart to thicken or stiffen - this is known as the left ventricular hypertrophy. When this happens, these changes make it difficult for the ventricle to properly distribute and pump blood to the body.

This condition heightens the risk of the individual to have a heart attack, for heart failure and sudden cardiac death. Remember that an aneurysm can happen anywhere in the body. Kidney artery aneurysm is a reality that could happen to somebody suffering from undetected and unmaintained high blood pressure. An aneurysm is a bulge in the wall of a person's blood vessel and may occur in an individual's kidneys as well.

When an aneurysm happens to an artery which leads up to the kidney this is known as a kidney artery aneurysm or a renal aneurysm. Atherosclerosis, which damages and weakens the artery wall, is one potential cause of this. As time passes, high blood pressure causes weakened arteries to enlarge and form a bulge which is an aneurysm. Aneurysms are dangerously fragile and can rupture, which leads to internal bleeding and can be life threatening to the patient.

Causes of High Blood Pressure

Dietary Factors

Contributing greatly to the increase of incidences of individual suffering from hypertension would be the ill habits they have gotten used to. Prevention and treatment of high blood pressure hinge largely on an individual's lifestyle choices which could contribute positively or negatively to a person's overall health.

Salt Restriction

The World Health Organization strongly recommends reducing salt intake to below 5 grams a day. This recommendation is to aid in the decrease of dangers of hypertension and health problems related to high blood pressure. Presently the average salt intake in almost all countries across the globe is between 5 grams to 12 grams a day. Lowering this number of average salt intake per day would greatly benefit people who are living with or without hypertension, but those who would benefit the most are individuals who do suffer from it.

Alcohol Consumption in Moderation

Raised high blood pressure and an increased susceptibility to stroke are linked to moderate to excessive consumption of alcoholic drinks. A drink a day for women and two for men are the recommended maximum number of alcoholic drinks the American Heart Association recommends, and no more. In this case, a drink would be:

- a 12 ounce (oz.) bottle of beer
- 1.5 oz. of 80-proof spirits
- 4 oz. of wine or 1 oz.
- 100-proof spirits

Should an individual find it difficult to cut back on drinking, it is best for them to be honest, upfront, and discuss this matter with their health care provider.

Less Fat, More Fruit and Vegetables

Patients who are at risk of and who already suffer from hypertension are strongly advised to up their intake of fruits and vegetables and minimize consumption of saturated and total fat.

Recommended Foods:
- High-fiber foods
- A variety of fruit and vegetables
- Beans

- Whole - Grain
- Omega - 3 rich fish twice a week
- Skinless poultry and fish
- Low-fat dairy products
- Pulses
- Nuts
- Non - tropical vegetable oils like an olive oil

It is crucial for a hypertensive patient to avoid trans-fats, or hydrogenated vegetable oils, as well as animal fats, wherever and whenever possible. Minding portion sizes is also strongly recommended.

Environmental Factors

There are indeed so many factors which contribute to high blood pressure and environmental factors are one of them. Factors in the environment of an individual's probability of acquiring hypertension would be temperature, time of day and changes in the climate. Sex, age and ethnicity also factor into this condition.

Activity and exercise (or lack of), extremity and body position, food, tobacco and alcohol intake and psychological stress are factors of behavior which contribute to blood pressure alteration.

A number of transient variables need to be controlled when a practitioner nurse measures and records a patient's blood pressure. Factors which can't be harnessed should be mindfully evaluated in order for the nurse practitioner not to make an wrong call or mistake the interpretation as an indication of pathology of the blood pressure changes.

Emotional Factors

When a patient is under duress or stress, this could cause the individual's blood pressure to temporarily increase. Now, it is important to know that having a routine and regular exercise regimen, about 30 minutes a day 3 - 5 times a week, can greatly reduce an individual's level of stress.

Doing activities to lower stress levels and manage anxiety can help improve one's health and this equates to a long term difference in lowering a person's blood pressure levels, most specially if a person has been diagnosed with high blood pressure. Although there is no proof yet that stress on its own brings about long term hypertension, it has been noted that stress is one of the factors which contribute to a person's decline in well - being. However it may also be that other factors like behavioral habits are linked to stress, such as drinking alcohol in excessive amounts, overeating and poor sleeping habits. It has also been reported that spikes in blood pressure which are short term stress-related may put an individual at risk of developing long term high blood pressure.

It has been noted that health conditions connected to stress like depression, anxiety, and isolation from family and friends may possibly have a link to heart disease. However there has been no evidence that gives resonance to these being related to long term high blood pressure. What it is instead that is suspected to damage one's arteries and leads to heart disease would be hormones a body produces when an individual is stressed emotionally.

Another matter to take note of would be destructive behavior which acts like fuel which feeds the fire, when a person is depressed. Depression can bring about destructive behavior in an individual like neglecting to ingest medication which helps curb and control high blood pressure or other cardiovascular conditions needing maintenance through medication.

Secondary Factors

High blood pressure is caused by other diseases in 10% of individuals who have this condition. This is called secondary hypertension - hypertension brought about by another illness. In these cases, treatment of the root cause is crucial. When the main problem is given attention and given treatment, blood pressure typically returns to normal or significantly lowers.

This 10% include conditions such as sleep apnea, tumors or other diseases of the adrenal gland, coarctation of the aorta - or narrowed aorta which a person is born with which can cause high blood pressure in the individual's arm, chronic kidney disease, the use of birth control pills, thyroid dysfunction, pregnancy, as well as illegal drugs and alcohol addiction. The other 90% of hypertension cases, known as primary hypertension is not known, although the cause specifically is yet unknown, it is determined that there are certain factors to consider and recognize as contributors to high blood pressure.

Signs and Symptoms of Hypertension

The danger of hypertension is that a person is usually oblivious to the fact that they have the condition. Statistically, almost one-third of people who have hypertension are not even aware that they have high blood pressure. The only way to figure out if a person is indeed hypertensive is through going in to see a physician and have regular, routine checkups. This is where genetics come into play; it is highly recommended for individuals who have family members who have the condition.

Should a person exhibit extremely high blood pressure consistently or more often than not, there are particular symptoms they would need to look out for which include, fatigue, confusion, severe headaches, difficulty in breathing, irregular heartbeats, pounding in the ear, chest or neck, and vision issues.

Chapter Three: How to Treat Hypertension

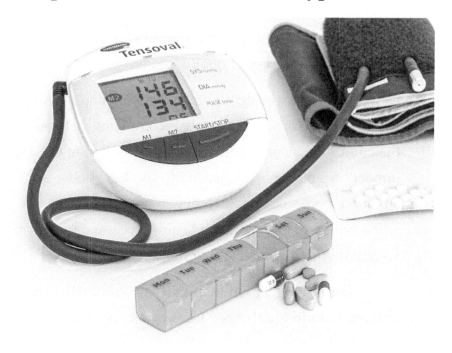

Even with medications given and prescribed by a physician, if a person does not make drastic changes to their lifestyle these medications are rendered useless and an additional expense - and quite a dent it will make to one's finances, it will! Here we shall discuss the importance of making wiser choices, and imposing self - discipline is crucial to leading a long and healthier existence. Your doctor may strongly recommend that you make several lifestyle changes which would include having a healthier diet with much less salt, also known as the Dietary Approaches to Stop Hypertension, or DASH, diet.

You would be given urgent advice to exercise regularly. If you are a smoker, then quitting smoking is another very strong recommendation you should heed to if you want to lead a better quality of life.

Do you have late nights of drinking and staying out late? Your doctor will definitely recommend that you limit the amount of alcohol you drink. Being heavyset has a great impact on a person's quality of life and how being so makes a person more susceptible to hypertension. Your physician will advise you to maintain a healthy weight or that you lose weight if you're overweight or obese.

In this chapter we shall find out about what changes in lifestyle individuals need to consider and make in order to lead a better quality of life and enjoy longevity. It is hoped that with the information here sheds light so that individuals suffering from this silent killer will be better armed and able to fend off this horrible malady which claims so many lives without warning.

Lifestyle Changes to Treat Hypertension

There are a number of ways to lower high blood pressure and the best way is a change in lifestyle. It seems easy enough but this method of improving one's health entails discipline and making mindful choices.

To be diagnosed with high blood pressure is not only a worrisome situation; it can be quite alarming as well. Not only is this situation another stressful situation for you but also for your family. Consider how it could have turned out if you hadn't found out sooner? You could have been in far worse straits.

The way you live and what you put into your body plays a large part on the quality of your life. Switching up your lifestyle does play an important role in treating a person's high blood pressure. If you listen to your physician and successfully control your blood pressure by leading a healthy lifestyle, you may just be able to avoid, delay or lessen the need for expensive, tiresome, daily medication.

Here are examples of lifestyle changes which can help you lower your risk of, control high blood pressure and lower your risks of heart disease without the use of medication:

Lose Those Extra Pounds and Watch Your Waistline

You might have thought that it was just a myth - watching your waistline, that is. But it isn't as studies show that keeping your weight down and watching that your waistline measurement doesn't go out of bounds is an important factor in keeping hypertension at bay. A person's blood pressure frequently increases when the weight of an individual increases. Being an overweight person can also cause interrupted breathing whilst you are asleep, which is known as Sleep Apnea; this condition will further promote the increase of an individual's blood pressure.

Shedding the pounds and losing weight is one of the most effective changes in a person's lifestyle to control blood pressure. To lose a mere 10 pounds or 4.5 kilograms doesn't only make a big difference in your road to a better quality of life; doing so can help reduce your blood pressure as well.

Aside from getting rid of the extra pounds, you should also generally keep a keen eye on your waistline. When a person carries too much weight around their waist, this can put them at greater risk of high blood pressure.

Generally, males are pegged as high risk if their waist measurement is more than 40 inches or 102 centimeters. Females, on the other hand, are classified as high risk for hypertension if their waist line measurement is over 35 inches or 89 centimeters. Talk to your physician about a healthy waist measurement for you as these numbers vary among ethnic groups.

Adapt a Regular Exercise Schedule

Make it a habit to have a regular regimen of exercise and active physical workouts of at least 30 minutes most days of the week. Doing so and maintaining this habit can decrease your blood pressure by a crucial 4 to 9 millimeters of mercury (mm Hg). It's vital to be consistent about keeping a routine exercise schedule because if you cease from exercising, your blood pressure can spike up again.

Should you have prehypertension, or a slightly high blood pressure, having an exercise regimen can aid you in averting the possibility of developing full blown hypertension. Now, if you are already hypertensive, regularly exercising can help lower your blood pressure to a safer, healthier level.

For someone who hasn't exercised in a while, it is best to start easy, but you need to mind that you do this religiously, otherwise changes will not happen. The best sorts of activities to help lower one's blood pressure include brisk walking, low-impact jogging, cycling, dancing and/or swimming. Another way to lose the weight and reduce blood pressure is strength training. Discuss and develop an exercise routine suitable for you, at this point, with your physician.

Mind What You Eat and Have A Healthier Diet

Switch up your diet and have one which is rich in fruits, vegetables, whole grains and low-fat dairy products. Skimp on cholesterol and saturated fats as doing so can help reduce your blood pressure by up to 14 mmHg - that makes a big difference! There is an eating plan you should ask your doctor about which is known as the DASH diet, short for Dietary Approaches to Stop Hypertension (DASH).

Changing your diet is admittedly not easy, but if you are mindful of the great changes it will benefit your quality of life, wouldn't you want to give yourself, and family, a better shot at living a life with optimal health?

Make it easier on yourself and adopt a healthy diet by keeping a journal of your food intake. It may seem anal at this time, but once you get used to doing so, it will get easier. Begin by writing down what you eat for the first week. This may give you enlightenment on your true eating habits. You will want to monitor what you consume, how much you eat, when you have it and the reason why. Again, it may sound tedious and ridiculous at first, but religiously keeping tabs on your food consumption will give you better insight as to what changes need to be done.

Potassium is a great way to reduce the effects of salt, or sodium, on your blood pressure, so consider upping your potassium intake at safe levels. Rather than taking over the counter potassium supplements, invest on fresh vegetables and fruits richly laden with potassium. Be sure to discuss potassium rich foods which would benefit you with your physician.

Learn the importance of being a smart shopper. Not only will this benefit you, but it will benefit your family as well. Make it a habit to read food labels and what components are in the foods you consider before making purchases. Eating at home not only does your finances well, but it gives you better control of what you put in your body.

Now, if there should be occasions when dining out is unavoidable, make sure that it is not considered a "cheat day" and stick to your new healthy eating plans.

Reduce the Sodium in Your Diet

Making even a slight reduction in salt intake will make a big difference to your health. Lessening the sodium in your daily diet can decrease your blood pressure by 2 to 8 mm Hg. This is a big deal if you quantify this reduction on a daily basis!

The effect of sodium intake on blood pressure is different amongst clusters of people. By and large, limiting sodium intake to less than 2,300 milligrams (mg) a day or less is the general recommendation. However, a lesser sodium intake of 1,500 mg a day or lower than that, is appropriately apt and encouraged for individuals with greater salt sensitivity.

These would be recommended for African-Americans (who historically, through extensive studies and observation, have a higher likelihood of developing hypertension), any individual whose age is 51 years old or older, any individual diagnosed with diabetes, chronic kidney disease, or high blood pressure.

Take note of these useful tips on how to decrease sodium in your diet:

- Read the labels of foods and find out about its sodium content. Processed foods have been one of the greatest culprits in recent times for the spike in individuals who suffer from hypertension. Choose low-sodium alternatives of beverages and food products you purchase when possible.

- Ingest less processed foods, if unavoidable. Cease eating processed foods if possible. Only a small amount of sodium is naturally in foods. Most of the sodium content in food is put in during processing.

- Avoid adding salt to your food when cooking at home. A mere 1 level teaspoon of salt has 2,300 mg of sodium. Consider use herbs or spices to add flavor to the food you cook as an alternative. If you are not confident about cutting out sodium in your diet then ease into it my reducing sodium slowly. This will allow your palate, over time, to get used to less sodium.

Limit and Monitor Your Alcohol Intake

Alcohol can be neither good nor bad for your health, largely depending on how much you drink. In small quantities, alcohol may potentially lower your blood pressure by 2 to 4 mm Hg. Another small step toward better health, right there! However, that protective effect is useless and considered as nothing if an individual drinks too much alcoholic beverages. Generally, the recommended alcohol intake (if unavoidable) is one alcoholic drink a day for females and for males older than 65 years old or more than two a day for men age 65 and below. One alcoholic beverage equates to 1.5 ounces of 80-proof liquor, five ounces of wine or 12 ounces of beer.

Having beyond the moderate quantities of alcoholic beverages can actually raise blood pressure by several alarming points. So beware, drinking more than the recommended alcohol intake can also reduce the instances of high blood pressure.

Stop Smoking

Each stick of cigarette a person smokes increases their blood pressure for quite a period of time after that fiery stub is crushed out. Ceasing smoking aids an individual's blood pressure to come back to normal levels. Individuals who stop smoking cigarettes, no matter what age they are, substantially increase their life expectancy aside from saving big bucks.

Cut Back on Caffeine and Caffeinated Drinks

How caffeine affects a person's blood pressure is still widely debated. Caffeine can elevate an individual's blood pressure by as much as 10 mm Hg for people who occasionally consume it, however there is little to no strong effect on blood pressure to individuals who habitually drink coffee. Even though the effects of regular and high amounts of caffeine ingestion on blood pressure aren't clear yet, the probability of a slight rise in blood pressure is real.

Is hypertension inherited?

Family members share behaviors, environments, lifestyles and more importantly genes, which play a big part in their wellness and health as well as their susceptibility for diseases. One condition which runs in the family is high blood pressure. The ethnicity and age of a person also comes into play.

Genetics and Family History

The process of heredity is when members of a family pass down traits from one generation to the next. The probability of heredity playing a role in family incidences with high blood pressure, heart disease and conditions related to them is very likely. On the other hand, families sharing a common environment as well as other probable factors increase that risk even more.

The dangers of developing high blood pressure within members of a family spikes up considerably when we combine heredity and unhealthy lifestyle habits such as excessive and frequent consumption of alcohol, smoking, leading a sedentary existence and an unhealthy diet.

It has been noted that high blood pressure is a disease which plagues the western world the most due to many factors such as unhealthy diets consisting of processed and high sodium content foods, almost no exercise, bearing great stress without relief and formed habits like excessive alcohol consumption and smoking. Most times, doctors are not able to determine the specific root cause of hypertension. This is what people in the medical field call essential hypertension. The lifestyle conditions above increase the risk of people developing this condition even more, as well as other factors like ethnicity and age.

Increasing the risk of hypertension in an individual is aging. As a person ages, the blood vessels toughen, and stiffen over time. There are about 65% adults who are over 60 years old and above who have developed high blood pressure according to medical experts and specialists.

Resistant Hypertension: Managing Tough High Blood Pressure

Should a person's high blood pressure be stubborn and remain high even though they are already taking different sorts of medicine usually a combination of 3 high blood pressure medications, then the person may have resistant hypertension.

Those with high blood pressure that are somewhat manageable but are taking varied kinds of high blood medication all at once (usually a minimum of four) just to manage the symptoms are also classified to have resistant hypertension. In these cases the probability of that their high blood pressure stems from a secondary medical condition is highly likely and must be considered.

Resistant hypertension doesn't mean that a person's blood pressure won't get lower. If your physician and you can determine the cause of your elevated blood pressure then there is a better chance for you to hit your target goal of lowering your blood pressure and get more effective treatment.

Your hypertension specialist or physician can make better evaluations on whether the drugs, and its doses, you are taking for hypertension is sufficient and appropriate for you. It will take some level of experimentation to figure out the best drugs and the proper dosages before you and your physician realize a good combination that works for you.

There are presently some therapies like electrical stimulation of carotid sinus baroreceptors and catheter-based radiofrequency ablation of renal sympathetic nerves that are recently making waves when it comes to treating hypertension. Aside from these new therapies, aldosterone antagonist like spironolactone (Aldactone) does frequently help to control resistant hypertension.

There are some medications, supplements or foods which can worsen high blood pressure or which may aid in preventing high blood pressure medications to work effectively. Should you be suffering from hypertension, it would be wise to be honest and upfront with your physician about other medications you may be taking and/or to discuss the lifestyle you lead.

If high blood pressure medication is not properly taken as directed by the physician, effectively is lost, and your blood pressure problems could worsen, and you would pay a bigger price for neglecting to heed advice of your specialist. Never change your treatment without consulting with your doctor. One's prescription, if you have gotten advice from others suffering from HBP, is not the same for all. Should you skip doses because you forgot, it's too expensive or it has side affects you feel, do not hesitate to discuss these with your physician in order to find better solutions. Some side effects of blood pressure medication can include diarrhea, headaches, unintentional weight loss, skin rash, dizziness, cough, and these tend to be minor.

Chapter Four: Managing Hypertension with Better Lifestyle

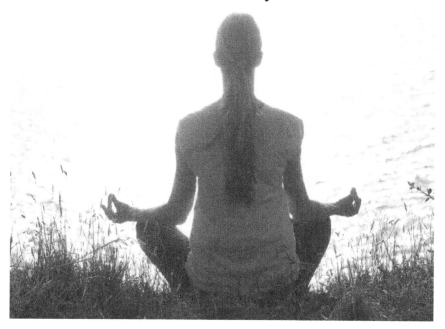

Whether male or female, both sexes can develop and are susceptible to high blood pressure. Other traits which you have no control over are factors like age and ethnicity which can also contribute to a person's tendency to develop high blood pressure. Blacks tend to develop high blood pressure more frequently than Hispanics, whites, Pacific Islanders, Asians, Alaska Natives, or American Indians. Compared to whites, blacks also develop high blood pressure earlier in life. Since blood pressure has a tendency to rise up as people get older, it only means that the risk for hypertension increases exponentially with age.

It is estimated that about nine out of ten Caucasians are likely to have hypertension during their lifetime. With the prevalence of processed foods and our mentality of quick fixes and fast answers, we've gotten used to having things happen immediately and fast results.

Aside from treatment, drugs and medication, a change in lifestyle choices will be discussed to you by your physician should they suspect you to be a likely candidate for hypertension. Since lifestyle plays a major role in the increasing prevalence of hypertension in the world today, many people have researched into finding other ways to manage and treat hypertension. Let's look into some of the other methods to controlling and managing hypertension in this chapter.

Exercise for Better Health and Eliminate Vices

It has been proven that people who are overweight or obese have a higher likelihood of developing high blood pressure and therefore have a more difficult time creating a better quality of life. Individual's with weight problems and have been diagnosed with high blood pressure have been advised by their physicians to take up exercising to decrease weight in order to have a better chance of having their medication and treatment to work better.

One need not go into exercising with a battle cry. It is best to work your way up to strength and endurance building rather than taking on too much too soon. After a while, exercising will come natural to you and you wouldn't even think twice about it. Set aside 30 minutes three to four times a week and make sure that you do not cheat yourself out of better health by skimping.

Minding a regular physical activity schedule is crucial to starting out any exercise regimen. Some of the recommended physical workouts advised by physicians would include brisk walking, cycling, low impact aerobic exercises, and swimming. As mentioned earlier, start out slow. No, this doesn't mean that you should move at a leisurely pace, instead what we mean by starting out slow is, doing exercises until you have produced enough sweat and feel that you have worked out. As you progress and lose the weight you will find yourself pushing yourself a little more are you reach peaks in your exercise times.

When going for walks, remind yourself to pick up the pace and watch your stance. So goes for all the other recommended exercises here. A person's blood pressure is elevated even after they have stubbed out their cigarette. Giving up cigarettes not only contributes to high blood pressure, it also is ta culprit of many other diseases which claim lives every year. Quitting smoking may seem like a

Mt. Everest challenge for some, but with the proper mindset, the willful support of family and friends, smoking can be eliminated as a habit for a person who has hypertension.

Others say that cutting down and slowly getting to a point of eliminating cigarettes worked for them, others report that cold turkey was how they successfully stopped huffing on that stick of tobacco. Either way, you will decide which is best for you. The important thing to remember is that smoking is one of the causes of hypertension and stopping now will only make you a healthier individual.

How to Manage Stress to control High Blood

Managing high blood pressure will only work if you take the necessary steps to curb this horrible silent killer. The benefits of leading a healthier lifestyle not only staves off hypertension, it will also give rise to an overall healthier you. Stress, although not ties in conclusively to hypertension, is an area of people's lives which is looked into and asked about by physicians because of the habits people form to "manage" stress. Due to stress, people have a tendency to binge eat, drink alcohol to excess, smoke and lead sedentary lives.

Couple all those ill-habits to deal with stress and aging, and then you have a perfect combination to be a candidate for high blood pressure. It has been observed that exercise generally reduces stress in people and allows them to think clearer and make wiser choices - possibly because they have invested effort, time and dedication which they wouldn't want to go to waste.

Benefits of Meditation

Meditation has been proven to be a simple and quick method to reduce stress. Meditation can wash away daily stress whilst bringing inner peace with it. If you are stressed and your everyday dealings have you anxious, worried and tense, do yourself a favor and consider meditation. If you spend even a few minutes in meditation, it can do wonders to restore calmness and inner peace.

This is a simple and inexpensive method which anyone can do. It is an activity that doesn't need fancy equipment or even a special location to do it. Whether you are walking, on the bus, waiting in line for your coffee or even in the middle of a great crowd of people, meditation is possible. Meditation in simple terms is just taking yourself to a "happy place", focusing on your breathing, and being in the moment.

It gives you a sense of balance, calm, and peace that can work wonders both for your emotional well-being and your overall health. The great thing about meditation is that these benefits don't end when you end your meditation session. Meditation helps you go about doing your usual work only more calmly. The best thing about it is that meditation could help you manage symptoms of certain medical conditions.

Do – It – Yourself Relaxation Techniques

Meditation could also be very useful especially if you have a medical condition, like hypertension, which is made worse by stress. As divided as researchers are about the benefits of meditation and even if they can't draw conclusions just yet of its benefits to health, there have been a great number of reports from individuals who have lauded this simple and inexpensive technique of channeling one's inner calm. Not only do they applaud meditation for lowering their everyday stress levels, many people have sworn to its efficiency on making them healthier individuals.

That being said, there have been research which suggests that meditation can possibly help people manage symptoms of conditions like asthma, cancer, chronic pain, anxiety, heart disease, high blood pressure, anxiety, depression, tension headaches, insomnia, and irritable bowel syndrome.

You want to discuss the pros and cons of meditation, should you be suffering from any of these conditions or other health issues, with your physician. Meditation isn't to be mistaken as a replacement for traditional medical treatment; however it can be a utilitarian addition to other treatments.

Types of Meditation

Meditation is basically a term for the numerous ways for a person to attain a relaxed state of mind. There are a number of methods and techniques for relaxation which carry components of meditation. All these methods are aimed at achieving an inner calm and peace.

Ways to meditate can include:

- Guided meditation, sometimes also called guided visualization or imagery, is a method of meditation where the person forms mental images of situations or places they find relaxing. This method of meditation uses as many senses as possible, like sights, smells, textures and sounds.

- Mantra meditation is a type of meditation, where the individual silently repeats or chants a calming word, phrase or thought to avoid getting distracted by their thoughts.

- Mindfulness meditation is a sort of meditation which is based on being mindful, or focusing on having a heightened awareness and acceptance of being in the moment. When a person practices mindfulness meditation, they broaden their conscious awareness. They zero in on what they are experiencing whilst meditating, such as the flow of their breath. During mindful meditation the individual can observe their thoughts and emotions, and release these thoughts without judgment.

- Qi gong is part of traditional Chinese medicine and is also a meditative practice which generally combines physical movement, meditation, relaxation, and breathing exercises which helps to restore and maintain balance.

- Tai chi is a gentle and graceful form of Chinese martial arts. When an individual practices tai chi, they perform a self-paced series of movements or postures in a slow, graceful way whilst focused on deep breathing.

- Transcendental meditation is a natural and simple technique wherein the individual silently repeats an assigned mantra, like a phrase, a word, or a sound, in a specific way. This sort of meditation could allow the person's body to settle into a state of profound rest and relaxation and their mind and thoughts to achieve a state of inner peace, with no need to concentrate or use up effort.

- Yoga is a series of postures and controlled breathing exercises which promote a calm mind and a more flexible body. As a person goes through poses which require concentration and balance, the individual is encouraged to focus less on anything else but the moment.

Chapter Five: How Diet Can Help You Fight Hypertension

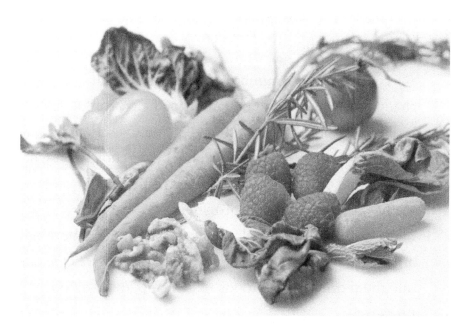

Making it a point to get better is something we owe ourselves and our loved ones. Creating an atmosphere which can allow us to live better lives is what we need to focus on if we expect to stick around for a while. Not only do we owe it to ourselves, but we owe it to our loved ones to not only be a role model for living healthier lives but also to inspire them to treat our bodies like temples and take care of it better.

Switching up from bad habits to good can be quite understandably challenging \but mindfulness and determination to live healthier can be attained if we just stop to consider the consequences if we continue to make the wrong health choices.

You've read it a number of times here about how lifestyle changes and getting rid of bad habits help promote better health and allow prescribed medication to work at its optimum level. Aside from making better choices on what we put into our bodies and getting treatment and medication from a health provider/specialist for hypertension, diet also plays a vital part in the betterment of an individual who suffers from this silent killer. Let's look into the recommended foods which help lower blood pressure.

Potassium and High blood Pressure

A key mineral that the body relies on heavily to function properly is potassium as it aids in reducing blood pressure levels by evening out the adverse effects of salt. Our kidneys function by way of controlling the amount of fluid which is stored in our bodies. Our kidneys work by filtering our blood and removing any extra fluids and it then stores it in our bladder turning it to urine. This is a process wherein sodium and potassium extracts the water from across the cell walls from our bloodstream and into a gathering channel which leads to the bladder. The more fluid retained in our bodies, the higher a person's blood pressure is.

Eating more fruits and vegetable will increase a person's level of potassium in their bodies and aid in resting this delicate balance. It will help a person's kidneys function as they efficiently and helps in lowering the blood pressure of an individual to a healthy level. But, do remember, that everything should be taken in moderation because it is possible that too much of a good thing become harmful to health. Make it a point not to overdose on potassium and choose natural foods instead of taking potassium supplements.

List of Potassium Rich Foods

We should all make it a point to eat, at a minimum, of at least five varied portions of vegetables and fruits each day to aid increase your potassium intake which helps in lowering blood pressure levels. A portion equates to about a fist-sized serving of fruits and vegetables or roughly 80 grams.

The following are amounts which represent a portion:

One medium-sized fruit	Banana, orange, apple or pear
Two small-sized fruits	Satsuma, apricots, plums
A slice of a large fruit	Pineapple. mango, melon
Two to three tablespoons	Grapes or berries
A glass (150ml)	Fresh fruit juice
One tablespoon	Dried fruit

The good news is that tinned fruits could be just as good as the fresh ones as long as you are mindful that these canned fruits don't have added fats, sugar or salt.

Keep in mind that all fruits and vegetables can help your body; however there are some fruits which contain more potassium than others. Some fruits which contain a high amount of potassium which are helpful in controlling and lowering blood pressure are apricots, bananas, orange juice, tomato puree or tomato juice, currants.

Make your fruit bowls even more effective in their job by cutting down (and hopefully, eventually eliminating) salt consumption. It may seem difficult to fathom that we would be able to cut down on salt, since we have been used to using it for cooking and seasoning our foods. But it is possible to marinade, season and make tasty dishes using very little of it and substituting salt by using herbs to add flavor to our dishes. Vegetables are also a good source of potassium, so make sure that you get your fresh greens, reds, purples, yellows and oranges in form of the vegetables we have listed below.

The following are amounts which represent a portion:

A dessert bowl	salad
Three heaping tablespoons	vegetables
Three heaping tablespoons	pulses like chickpeas, beans, lentils and the like
A glass (150ml)	vegetable juice

Again, canned or frozen vegetables work just as well as the fresh ones as long as you watch out for any added fats, sugar and/or salt, because you should really be avoiding those.

Keep in mind, that all vegetables help make you become healthier and aid your body, but some have more potassium in them than others. Some vegetables that are particularly rich in potassium and could help in lowering blood pressure levels are sweet potatoes, asparagus, cabbage, potatoes, spinach, and sprouts. We want to remind you again that the effect of all these potassium rich foods will only work if you mindfully avoid the intake of salt.

Apart from fruit and vegetables, there are other ways that you can increase the amount of potassium in your diet, and which supply your body with a boost of helpful vitamins and minerals. There are other foods which are laden with potassium and help in the lowering of blood pressure levels. Apart from the fruits and vegetables mentioned previously, tuna is also a good source of potassium.

Some foods which are specifically rich in potassium and can be more helpful in controlling blood pressure would be salmon, fat-free milk, macadamia nuts, mushrooms, wheat germ, tuna (but not in brine as this just cancels out the effectiveness of potassium intake because of the salt content), yoghurt, eggs, almonds, bran, whole meal and pasta. Don't forget to cut down on the quantity of salt you eat or none of the health measures you take will be effective.

Benefits of Miracle Foods

If you've been searching for other beneficial foods to help lower your blood pressure level, then search no further as we have compiled a list of great eats available to you and probably already in your refrigerator which you can take to aid in treating hypertension. Let's take a look at some beneficial foods and how adding these in your diet each day helps stave off and decrease blood pressure levels.

Can Celery Drop hypertension in 1 week?

High blood pressure has become a big health issue for many people all over the world. According to statistics from various health organizations, in America alone, there are around 76 million Americans suffering from hypertension.

The compound 3-n-butylphthalide or phthalide is found in celery juice that also adds to the vegetable's overall taste. When this chemical enters the body phthalide helps relax and smoothen the muscles in the blood vessel's walls. Blood pressure goes down as it allows blood flow easily because the vessels have been dilated already.

Garlic and Onion Benefits

Garlic has historically been lauded to be one of the best home remedies to treat and lower blood pressure. It has powerful antioxidants such as allicin, selenium and Vitamin C which are very effective in thinning the blood and make the arteries flexible. This wonder veggie also promotes and stimulates the production of nitric oxide in the body which in turn increases smooth blood flow throughout a person's body.

For garlic to work best on a hypertensive individual, a person would need to swallow or chew a few cloves of raw garlic, every day on an empty stomach. Beware that you don't overdo it as consuming too much raw garlic may cause side effects and skin rashes.

Onions have a flavonoid component called quercetin, which can also be found in apple skins, and is a very effective food source to lower cholesterol, promote weight loss, protects from heart disease and allow for a smoother blood flow in a person's system, hence, lowering blood pressure. One leading cause of hypertension, atherosclerosis, is prevented by the components found in onions just like garlic, onions work at its finest in preventing hypertension when eaten raw.

How Oatmeal Can Work Wonders

Oatmeal is a fantastic breakfast or snack choice if a person has high blood pressure. However, oat bran is better able in providing even more health benefits, because it has higher fiber content which aids in lowering blood pressure as it improves digestive health. Oatmeal and oat bran are low-sodium foods which can be prepared as a hot cereal topped off with fruit and can be used in pancakes.

How Water Can Fight Hypertension

Drinking sufficient quantities of water is, one of the healthiest, most affordable, and really effective method which helps lower a person's blood pressure. Continued and prolonged dehydration causes blood vessels to tighten and constrict, which gives way for the body to retain water. It restricts and reduces water loss via urination, perspiration, and respiration. The bad news is, constricted blood vessels will instruct the heart to labor harder, resulting in a rise in blood pressure. Many of us have heard of and been advised about the eight-glasses-a-day rule, and still don't abide by it. However, for a more tailor-fit approach, divvy up your body weight in two. The result or sum of that, in ounces is the ideal water amount a person should be the minimum target to consume per day, For example, a 150-pound person should shoot for at least 75 ounces daily.

Fish Oils to Keep Your Arteries Healthy

The different functions of fish oil work to reduce or decrease plaque from forming in the arteries and lower the risk of heart disease. Using these oils reduce the quantity of LDL in building up as plaque. Lessening the inflammation on the walls of the blood vessel also lessens the number of platelets which build up at the site to repair it, and in turn decreases the danger of clot formation.

Clots are able to break free and get lodged in arteries, decreasing vital blood flow to the heart. This incident can cause heart attack or a stroke. When bloods vessels are dilated they have less of a chance of being blocked by plaque. When a person gets enough omega-3 to omega-6 fatty acid portions, this increases prostacyclin, which lessens platelet production and lowers arterial spasms.

Dietary Reminders for People with High Blood

To recap what we've discussed in this chapter, an individual diagnosed with high blood pressure is to lessen, if not eliminate, salt intake. If this is not followed, everything else an individual does (like taking medication) will be useless and cancelled out.

Limit alcohol consumption and get help if not able to do it on your own. Drinking alcohol in excess promotes hypertension and negates other positive changes one makes in their lifestyle if alcohol is not cut down drastically. Double up on a healthy diet and stay away from saturated fats, sugars and most especially salt. Get plenty of potassium (if you can't help having a dash or two of salt with your meals) because potassium helps balance out the sodium in the cells of the body. Remember the DASH diet and abide by it.

Chapter Six: Unconventional Treatments for Hypertension

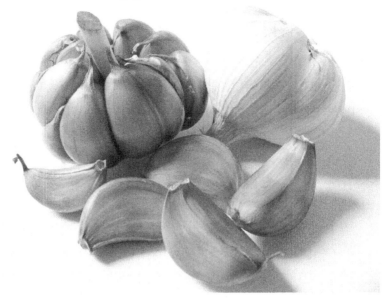

High blood pressure increases the chances of a person to have a stroke, a heart attack or kidney problems. So it comes as no surprise that many individuals with this condition are interested in taking hold of and controlling hypertension. The side effects with are brought about by antihypertensive drugs can be expensive and troublesome for some people and they search for alternatives.

The good news about getting back on the road to being healthy after being diagnosed with hypertension or high blood pressure is that there are a number of ways to stave off and keep hypertension at bay or completely eradicate it from a person's life. Through years of observation, experimentation and successful results, complementary treatments to make one live a better quality of life are available these days.

You have read about healthy diet and exercise to be some of the key factors which aid in treating or even getting rid of high blood pressure. Aside from these, recent studies have revealed that complementary and alternative medicines can aid in lowering blood pressure levels of a person successfully.

Let's take a look at how CAM (Complementary and Alternative Medicines are able to lower, reduce and aid in blood pressure problems. You want to remember that as with anything outside of the medical realm, you want to discuss these alternative methods with your physician before trying out anything on your own. Just because it worked for a friend, it doesn't necessarily mean it would for you as some herbal medicines can contradict medications you may already be taking.

Herbal Medicines

Benefits of Gingko Biloba

Ginkgo has components which improve blood flow and decrease inflammation. Ginkgo biloba also acts as an antioxidant and protects the cells from damage. Presently, ginkgo is possibly best known for its potential to improve memory. It is also taken to treat all sorts of blood-flow disorders. Aside from all these benefits, ginkgo biloba is also used against mental decline in adults with dementia. Recent research now focuses on standardizing ginkgo extract, which is highly concentrated.

Benefits of Hawthorn

Despite the fact that hawthorn has not been looked into specifically in individuals with high blood pressure, there are some people who think its benefits in treating heart disease may also apply to treating high blood pressure or hypertension. But there isn't enough research to tell for sure whether hawthorn is effective in decreasing blood pressure.

In one research, hawthorn extract was determined to be effective for hypertension in patients with type 2 diabetes and who were taking prescribed medicines as well.

Patient-participants were given to take 1,200 mg of hawthorn extract every day or placebo for 16 weeks. Those who took hawthorn had reduced blood pressure compared to those who took the placebo. Again, it is highly advisable and recommended that you discuss this with your physician before taking anything on your own.

Benefits of Maitake Mushroom

Maitake mushroom can decrease blood pressure though it may not be equally effective for everyone. Ingesting maitake could make a patient's blood pressure become too low which is why it should be taken with prescribed medication as well.

Maitake mushroom could raise the blood thinning effects of Coumadin and possibly increase the chances of bleeding. The physician may have to closely monitor the patient's blood pressure levels upon maitake mushroom intake, and the dosage of warfarin medication should also be monitored because it may need changes upon intake. The proper dose of maitake mushroom hinges on a few factors like the patient's age, some other conditions, and overall effect on the body. Presently, there isn't sufficient scientific information to confirm an appropriate range of doses for maitake mushroom.

Remember that products like this may depend on how the body responds, proper dosage is also very important. Remember that it is imperative that you talk to your healthcare provider before taking anything outside of what is prescribed to you.

Benefits of Olive Leaf Extract

The ancient Egyptians used extracts from the olive leaf for purposes of curing and other medicinal purposes. Nowadays researchers confirm the health benefits of the olive leaf and how it serves in many ways. One of these benefits includes its usefulness to fight against heart disease, high cholesterol and as an active supplement to lower high blood pressure. Scientist has recently discovered the awesome ability of the potent olive leaf to lessen blood pressure and cholesterol.

Benefits of Reishi Mushroom

Careful studies have shown that extracts from the reishi mushroom can lessen high blood pressure to a significant degree. This was proven effective even in patients who did not respond to conventional antihypertensive drugs. Studies conducted on animals revealed that reishi mushroom extract lowers blood pressure through a central inhibition of nerve activity; however it typically doesn't slow down the heart rate or induce a sedative effect. Reishi mushroom extract also has a mild to moderate effect on lowering platelet production, which could further aid in decreasing the risk of cardiovascular disease.

Ayurvedic Medicine

Ayurvedic treatment for hypertension is targeted to identify the primary cause of the condition and then administer herbs which can eliminate the condition from its source. In order for this to transpire, it is crucial that digestion is improved. The toxins which have built up in the heart channels must be eradicated. Finally, mind relaxation techniques which include meditation, pranayama and yoga are then recommended for the patient to make sure that the mind stays calm and stable.

Traditional Chinese Medicine

Traditional Chinese medicine (TCM) has a unique outlook about high blood pressure. In TCM, it is thought that the body wants balance. A sound body is an individual's natural state and any sort of malady or health issue is traced back to something in the body which is out of balance. Chinese medicine works hard to bring every patient back into balance so as to have better health. High blood pressure is fatal if not detected early and managed, however a more positive outlook is that high blood pressure is a big red flag that something in a person's lifestyle needs swift changing.

From the viewpoint of Traditional Chinese Medicine hypertension is a sign that there is an abnormality which indicated there is a part of the body which is under-regulated caused by a number of factors. TCM blames continued stress, a sedentary lifestyle, organ damages, an unhealthy diet all play in contributing to raised blood pressure levels.

TCM has fewer side effects and and has greater advantages in treating hypertension and symptoms related to it. TCM wouldn't be considered to work as quickly as conventional medical treatments but it does reduce the risk of complications. It focuses on holistic health care and when integrated with conventional Western treatments, both these have better and more favourable results. Most times, mild to moderate cases of hypertension are treated with success with just TCM.

Detoxification

Lowering high blood pressure is vital because if left untreated it will become extremely dangerous. High blood pressure could be the outcome of way too much stress, abusively high alcohol consumption, an extremely poor diet, obesity, abusive consumption of stimulants. It could also be attributed to heavy metal toxicity, smoking, lack of or absence of physical activity and exercise. It could result from an underlying disease, magnesium deficiency or a combination of a number of these.

One terrific detoxification method is exercise. Exercise does not only lessen blood pressure, it also makes an individual sweat out toxins which could cause high blood pressure primarily. Another detox recommendation is to get flax into a person's diet. This is a heart-healthy food which encourages healthy bowel movements, which in turn makes it easier to pass toxins out of the body. The patient also has to learn and practice breathing exercises, which will allow them to dispel the chemicals in their body through breath.

Chapter Seven: First Aid Treatments for High Blood Pressure

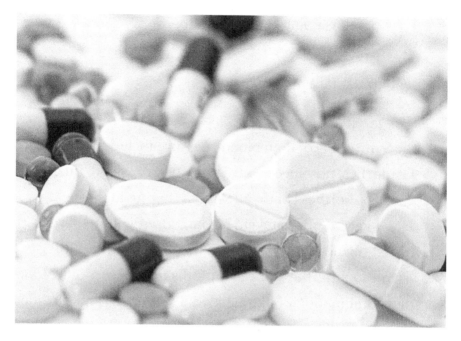

It is almost surprising to know that essential hypertension is almost unknown in developing countries, with no rise in blood pressure because of advancing age. It would lead one to the belief that over 90% of blood pressure conditions are directly related to Western lifestyle and diet. Missing doses of blood pressure medication can lead to renal failure, stroke, heart failure, eclampsia and preeclampsia when the patient is pregnant. Needless to say, it is vital to be able to tell if a person is going through an episode of hypertension attack the soonest. However, most of the time there are really no visible signs or physical symptoms either.

The most important thing to remember is to go get a medical checkup the soonest a person feels off or unwell. Let's find out more about how to identify if a family member or yourself is going through a hypertensive attack.

Symptoms of Hypertension Attack

Symptoms of high blood pressure include dizziness, headaches, nosebleeds, sweating, blurry vision, flushed cheeks, shortness of breath, and a ringing in the ears. However, it is probable to be diagnosed with hypertension and show no symptoms at all. Most of the time, HBP is asymptomatic but some symptoms may be any one of these or a combination of lightheadedness, vertigo and dizziness, severe chest pain, shortness of breath, tinnitus, seizures, severe anxiety, loss of consciousness, severe headache, nausea and vomiting, fainting episodes, memory loss, personality changes, trouble concentrating, irritability or progressive loss of consciousness and other symptoms related to a secondary condition.

These symptoms can be nonspecific and don't always indicate hypertension as a cause. However, first aid training courses must express the importance of the value of measuring blood pressure in individuals who claim to be having these symptoms. A handheld electronic blood pressure monitor can be used to determine this. Before taking a person's blood pressure the patient must rest for at least 20 minutes. The patient has to be seated or lying down. Use a correct sized blood pressure cuff and slip it onto the upper arm at the level of heart.

First Aid Treatment

- Be certain that the blood pressure reading is accurate most especially if the patient shows no symptoms like headache or chest pains.

- Have the patient relax. Calm the patient by instructing them to focus on their breathing and have them breathe slowly and deeply. There are times when slow breathing can lower the blood pressure.

- Should the patient have maintenance drugs prescribed to them for high blood pressure, have them take it.

- Give the patient high blood pressure medicines if the following circumstances are present: If the blood pressure is above 140/90 and the patient shows symptoms like headache, dizziness, or chest pains and if the blood pressure is 160/100 or above.

- The common first aid medication physicians give to reduce the blood pressure include one tablet of Clonidine 75 mcg to be taken orally or one tablet of Captopril 25 mg, also to be taken orally. These tablets can also be placed, to be dissolved, under the tongue for quicker action. For most cases, taking them orally will suffice. Consult with physician first.

- Remember that not all cases of high blood pressure have to be given medications. There are times when external causes of high blood pressure like anger, tension or pain is to blame. Make sure to identify if this is the case. Finally, see your doctor for a check-up.

Chapter Eight: Hypertension and Associated Diseases

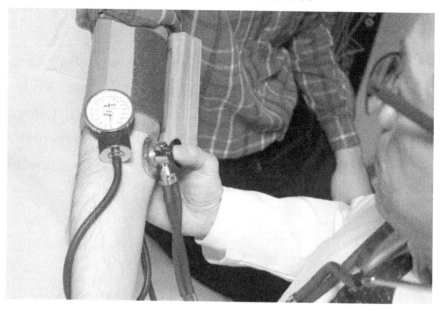

It is but wise to get regular and routine checkups with your physician if you suspect yourself or a family member to have high blood pressure. Keep in mind that high blood pressure is not a condition limited only to the aging population; it can also make victims of the younger set. With lifestyle choices and environmental conditions to consider, hypertension is becoming more and more prevalent in this day and age due to choices we make or possibly from another medical condition. Either way, it is best to see your doctor whether you think you are in the pink of health or, most especially so, if you are displaying any of the symptoms previously discussed here. Hypertension can be a sign of other diseases present in the body which can go undetected. As we previously learned, traditional Chinese medicine sees hypertension as a signal that there has been an imbalance in the body, hence, if caught early, it is an opportunity to set things right.

Individuals with high blood pressure typically show no symptoms; therefore patients can be suffering silently with the condition for years and not even know it. Other underlying causes could also be the culprit for hypertension, hence it is crucial to get medical checkups on a routine basis.

Associated Diseases

Below are the common illnesses that have been associated with hypertension. Treatments for these diseases are much more complicated since the medicines prescribed could also have side effect to the current medical condition of a patient.

Cardiovascular Diseases

The heart supplies, pumps and carries blood throughout the entire body. Over time, uncontrolled high blood pressure will damage the heart in several ways and can be a risky health deterrent for the individual.

Coronary artery disease causes damage to the arteries. These arteries serve as the channel so that blood can flow to the heart muscle. Arteries which are toughened and blocked by coronary artery disease eventually lead heart ailments. When this happens, the blood can't flow as it freely should to the heart. A person can also have chest pain, arrhythmias (irregular heartbeats) or heart attack.

An enlarged left heart can be caused by hypertension. This happens when high blood pressure pushes the heart to pump more supply of blood to the rest of the individual's body making it work harder. These changes almost prevent the ventricle to do its job of pumping blood to the body. This creates a condition which puts the individual at risk for various heart ailments, failure and even sudden cardiac arrest.

Over time, these arterial heart problems due to high blood pressure can make the heart muscle become overworked and function a lot less efficiently. Eventually, the overwhelmed heart just starts to wear out, falter and completely stop functioning. Damage from heart attacks exacerbates this problem.

Kidney Diseases

Hypertension is one of the most typical causes of renal failure. This is because HBP can damage both the large arteries and the glomeruli or the tiny blood vessels found in the kidneys. When damaged, the kidneys can't filter waste from the blood effectively; this will then result to dangerous levels of toxic waste in the body which can affect other organ functions, once this happens, the patient may likely end up with dialysis (to help filter waste out the blood) or kidney transplantation.

Glomerulosclerosis is a kind of kidney damage that is caused by the scarring of the tiny blood vessels which filter fluid and waste from the blood. Glomerulosclerosis can render the kidneys near useless and will be unable to clean out the blood, which will eventually lead to kidney failure.

Kidney artery aneurysm is a blocked out artery that causes problems in the blood pathway leading to the kidney. One possible culprit is atherosclerosis because it damages the artery wall. High blood pressure in an artery can cause a part in the kidney to enlarge and form a bulge (aneurysm) which can rupture and lead to fatal and severe internal bleeding.

Aneurysm

The constant pressure of blood moving through a weakened artery, over time, can cause a part of the artery wall to enlarge and create an aneurysm. An aneurysm (or a bulge) has the potential to rupture and become life-threatening because of internal bleeding. Aneurysms can cluster in any artery anywhere in the body, but are most common in the body's biggest artery called the aorta.

Dementia

Dementia is a brain disease which results in challenges and issues with memory, thinking, reasoning, speaking, movement and vision. There are several reasons for dementia. Vascular dementia is one cause and can occur because of the narrowing and blockage of the arteries which is responsible for supplying blood to the brain. This can also occur because of strokes which are caused by an interruption of blood flow to the brain. In both cases, high blood pressure could be the culprit.

Sexual Dysfunction

As men age, the inability to get and keep an erection, medically termed as erectile dysfunction becomes more common when males reach their 50th year. Erectile dysfunction is likelier to become more apparent if the aging male also has high blood pressure. High blood pressure, over time, causes damages to the lining of the man's blood vessels causing their arteries to toughen, become inflexible and become narrow (medically termed as atherosclerosis). Atherosclerosis is a disease of the arteries which is characterized by plaque deposits of fatty material in the inner walls of the artery and results to a limited blood flow.

For men, this equates to less blood flow to the penis. For several men, lesser blood flow makes it challenging to get and maintain an erection. This problem is fairly typical especially amongst men who have not been treating their high blood pressure.

Women too may experience sexual dysfunction as a result and side effect of high blood pressure. High blood pressure may lessen blood flow to the vagina. For several women, this can lead to a decline in sexual desire and/or arousal. This can also cause vaginal dryness, or challenges in achieving orgasm. Improving arousal and lubrication can help. Like men, women can experience anxiety and relationship issues due to sexual dysfunction.

Index

C

D

I

J

K

L

M

T

U

V

W

Photo Credits

Page 2 Photo by user karlneo via Pixabay.com, https://pixabay.com/en/medical-girl-health-2414782/

Page 13 Photo by user Army Medicine via Pixabay.com, https://www.flickr.com/photos/armymedicine/5805435297/

Page 31 Photo by user StockSnap via Pixabay.com, https://pixabay.com/en/people-man-guy-frustration-2568886/

Page 43 Photo by user stevepb via Pixabay.com, https://pixabay.com/en/hypertension-high-blood-pressure-867855/

Page 58 Photo by user Pexels via Pixabay.com, https://pixabay.com/en/meditate-meditation-peaceful-1851165/

Page 68 Photo by user dbreen via Pixabay.com, https://pixabay.com/en/carrot-kale-walnuts-tomatoes-1085063/

Page 80 Photo by user Gadini via Pixabay.com, https://pixabay.com/en/garlic-purple-garlic-head-of-garlic-618400/

Page 89 Photo by user stevepb via Pixabay.com, https://pixabay.com/en/headache-pain-pills-medication-1540220/

Page 94Photo by user Alterfines via Pixabay.com, https://pixabay.com/en/medicine-patient-doctor-voltage-2361046/

References

"6 Drinks That Lower Blood Pressure" HealthUnlocked.com

https://healthunlocked.com/diabeteshelp/posts/1158566/6-drinks-that-lower-blood-pressure

"8 Effective Home Remedies for High Blood Pressure" FindHomeRemedy.com

http://www.findhomeremedy.com/8-effective-home-remedies-for-high-blood-pressure/

"Can Fish Oil Reverse Plaque in Arteries" Livestrong.com

http://www.livestrong.com/article/466377-can-fish-oil-reverse-plaque-in-arteries/

"Causes of High Blood Pressure" Webmd.com

http://www.webmd.com/hypertension-high-blood-pressure/guide/blood-pressure-causes#1

"Causes of Secondary Hypertension"

Webmd.com

http://www.webmd.com/hypertension-high-blood-pressure/guide/secondary-hypertension-causes#1

"Checking Your Blood Pressure at Home" Cleveland Clinic

https://my.clevelandclinic.org/health/articles/checking-your-blood-pressure-at-home

"Chinese Medicine Guideline for Hypertension Management" Shen-Nong.com

http://www.shen-nong.com/eng/lifestyles/tcm_hypertension_chinese_medicine_guideline.html

"Difference between High Blood Pressure and Low Blood Pressure" DifferenceBetween.info

http://www.differencebetween.info/difference-between-high-blood-pressure-and-low-blood-pressure

"Environmental and behavioral factors that can affect blood pressure" NCBI.NLM.NIH.GOV

https://www.ncbi.nlm.nih.gov/m/pubmed/4069459/

"Family History and Other Characteristics That Increase Risk for High Blood Pressure" Cdc.gov

https://www.cdc.gov/bloodpressure/family_history.htm

"First Aid Management of Hypertensive Crisis" FirstAidSaskatoon.com

http://firstaidsaskatoon.ca/first-aid-management-of-hypertensive-crisis/#ixzz4oyW6C4cB

"Intro Into Mechanics" Beat Blood Pressure

https://beatbloodpressure.wordpress.com/2011/02/09/intro-into-mechanics/

"Hawthorne" University of Maryland Medical System

http://www.umm.edu/health/medical/altmed/herb/hawthorn

"Hypertension" Jiva.com

https://www.jiva.com/diseases/hypertension/

"Hypertension" Wikipedia

https://en.m.wikipedia.org/wiki/Hypertension

"Lose the Salt, Not the Flavor" Everyday Health

https://www.everydayhealth.com/hypertension-pictures/lose-the-salt-not-the-flavor.aspx

"Maitake Mushroom" RxList.com

http://www.rxlist.com/maitake_mushroom-page3/supplements.htm

"Masked Hypertension: A Review" Nature.com

http://www.nature.com/hr/journal/v30/n6/abs/hr200763a.html?foxtrotcallback=true

"Meditation: A simple, fast way to reduce stress" MayoClinic.org

http://www.mayoclinic.org/tests-procedures/meditation/in-depth/meditation/art-20045858

"Reishi and High Blood Pressure" Healing Reishi

https://healingreishi.wordpress.com/reishi-high-blood-pressure/

"What causes high blood pressure?" Healthline.com

http://www.healthline.com/health/high-blood-pressure-hypertension#causes3

"White Coat Hypertension: 6 Things to Know" BerkeleyWellness.com

http://www.berkeleywellness.com/self-care/preventive-care/article/white-coat-hypertension-6-things-know

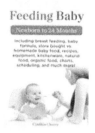

Feeding Baby
Cynthia Cherry
978-1941070000

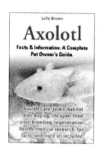

Axolotl
Lolly Brown
978-0989658430

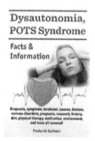

Dysautonomia, POTS
Syndrome
Frederick Earlstein
978-0989658485

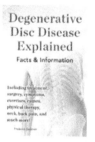

Degenerative Disc
Disease Explained
Frederick Earlstein
978-0989658485

Sinusitis, Hay Fever,
Allergic Rhinitis Explained
Frederick Earlstein
978-1941070024

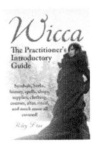

Wicca
Riley Star
978-1941070130

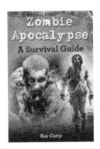

Zombie Apocalypse
Rex Cutty
978-1941070154

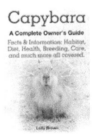

Capybara
Lolly Brown
978-1941070062

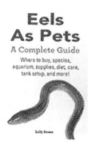

Eels As Pets
Lolly Brown
978-1941070167

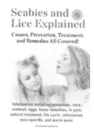

Scabies and Lice Explained
Frederick Earlstein
978-1941070017

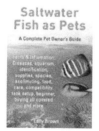

Saltwater Fish As Pets
Lolly Brown
978-0989658461

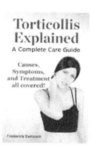

Torticollis Explained
Frederick Earlstein
978-1941070055

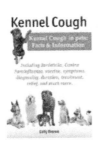

Kennel Cough
Lolly Brown
978-0989658409

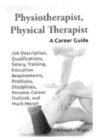

Physiotherapist, Physical
Therapist
Christopher Wright
978-0989658492

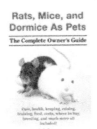

Rats, Mice, and Dormice
As Pets
Lolly Brown
978-1941070079

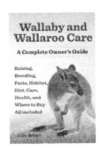

Wallaby and Wallaroo Care
Lolly Brown
978-1941070031

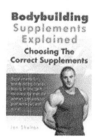

Bodybuilding Supplements
Explained
Jon Shelton
978-1941070239

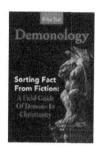

Demonology
Riley Star
978-19401070314

Pigeon Racing
Lolly Brown
978-1941070307

Dwarf Hamster
Lolly Brown
978-1941070390

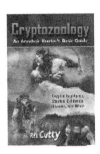

Cryptozoology
Rex Cutty
978-1941070406

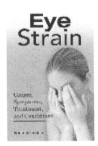

Eye Strain
Frederick Earlstein
978-1941070369

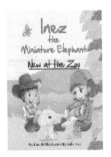

Inez The Miniature Elephant
Asher Ray
978-1941070353

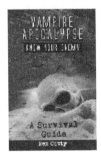

Vampire Apocalypse
Rex Cutty
978-1941070321

Made in the USA
Monee, IL
11 July 2023

38957939R00069